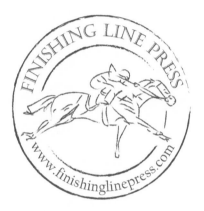

Mind Lit in Neon

poems by

R.J. Lambert

Finishing Line Press
Georgetown, Kentucky

Mind Lit in Neon

Publisher: Leah Huete de Maines
Editor: Christen Kincaid
Cover Art: Loui Jover
Author Photo: R.J. Lambert
Cover Design: Elizabeth Maines McCleavy

Order online: www.finishinglinepress.com
also available on amazon.com

Author inquiries and mail orders:
Finishing Line Press
P. O. Box 1626
Georgetown, Kentucky 40324
U. S. A.

Table of Contents

*

*

One must imagine Sisyphus happy.

BLAISE PASCAL

Feedback Loop

Here I go again. Can't help myself
from noticing a comma isn't there.
I read a missing pause as lack of listening.

Listen, some men are serial offenders.
Didn't he hear me say, "Don't
throw your phone at me." "Don't
break another glass." There is both
a grammar & a proper name for objects.
Sometimes a "glass" is not a "goblet."

"But what's a goon to a goblin?"
When Weezy was Dwayne, he may
have heard a mother say, "Out there,
you're some big man." "But to me, OG,
you will always be a little boy."

What you picture when you hear "kid gloves"
is generational. Imagine fingers tucked in satin.
Each ear pierced by metal, rung with pearls.

How "breakfast at Tiffany's" was an action
before a book adapted to a movie
hooked inside a song. How a blue
box is one person's everything,
but, for most of us, nothing at all.
The opposite of "affinity" is "avidity."

There is both a color & an odor
for things. As a boy I learned blood
has a smell. Cooking out, dad clipped
his middle finger off. The finger fell mute
from its hand. "F—you," it no longer said to life.
"Take my wife & leave me the guitar."

Imagine a finger having its own story. Imagine
having been allowed, briefly, inside

another person. Imagine having borne the ring.

In a car named after Saturn my mom
mentioned lightly how marriage crumbles
under the gravity of a ketchup bottle.
Ketchup, catsup—here I go again.
Condemned to quibble over condiments.
Imagine the tomatoes ringing the linoleum.

I keep the fridge & microwave wiped clean.
My stepdad doesn't stand for counter crumbs.
I only sometimes tuck the sheets. Before me,
the shower knob acquainted someone else's thumb.

Imagine I told my doctor, "Enough
with all the labs." "The virus is here to stay."
"My health is more or less the same as yesterday."
This metaphor for blood is visceral.
What's a demon to a hemoglobin?

I remember my first ambulance.
Play paused like a baby's breath upstairs.
We had chased all day & laughed
out loud. Imagine the medic, "I'm sorry,
ma'am." "We see SIDS all the time."
"Please don't ring us with your panic."

Here I go again. Taking the breaking
personal. Projecting names
at somewhat shattered things.
A synonym for "mundanity" is "divinity."

Imagine me, begging you to listen.
Instructed to unornament my urgency.
Tell me, again, how must my griefs be boxed.

What was the best day of your life?

It was a night.

BRIGITTE BARDOT

Future Tense

I see it coming,
blue, like a train.
The chassis
slips over
in shadow
& burns
awhile under
the sun.
The engine
hums, chews
syllables,
swallowing
whole letters
wholly.
Such things
change lives,
leave halves
behind
as questions
without asking.
Do I have nothing
left but "why"?
"Why" pauses.
"Why" scorches
letters. A
slow coal burn
narrows
in the throat
like traffic down
a one-way
street.

Cruise Control

Downthedrivefromtown

the lake that dried to ground
over the summer freezes

what it thaws each day. In bed
tonight I eye the raft

of ducks that kick through floes
to open floating holes.

Sleep's long frictions emphasize
that what I must retain from day

to day is froze in the abstract
ion wakefulness prevents again

st. So much so, sleep breaks
my body braces ice my skin

brightwhitefromunderwaterlights.

Mr. Liquor Delivers

people telling me the same
thing that I need
to go & stop

worrying when
the bomb comes
along I guess

no bad news is
a kind of good news is
just another shadow

whispering persistently
to seek a substance
& a sugar

like a question
mark grinding
a sweet care

lessness
not it that has
not even it a little

Fight, Flight, Freeze

My verbs start wanting
more stresses,
some nouns to be held,

some little preposition.
In short, my sounds
are out of practice.

My words are not
infinite, my word is
what's lacking.

The answer is fractured
from asking. A "but"
holds back the "ifs" & "ands"

& utters nothing.
Sometimes the silence
sounds like sirens.

Sometimes the quiet
conjugates me
like a verb.

Habits of Creature

My inner, my outer, my over & under.
My thinner & fatter. My lightning,

my thunder. My days & my nights
& my mids & my noons.

My suns, my stars, my phases
of moons. My waters:

my rivers & oceans & seas. My
valley of deserts, my mountain of trees.

My mother, my father, my sister, my killer.
A thunder rolls over. A river of shivers.

Abated at bottom, so long
from the top. Some fruit on the floor.

A bucket. A mop. The fog
on the windows & prints

on the dresser. The best,
now the worst. The greater, the lesser.

The TV & phone & the speakers
connected. The cats & the plants &

the dishes neglected.
The neighbors are talking

& calling me back. The thicker
the fog, the looser the slack.

Today to tomorrow, when never
is now, for whether whomever

whatever allows. Speaking out sparks
friendly fire inside. We run. We jump.

You seek & I hide. The why of the try
is a promise unspoken. My heart,

like a record or dream,
being broken. A call or a text

or a visit would do, or forever
regret what I never with you.

The long & the short of farewell is
"go slow." My follow will after

wherever you go. My honest, my truth,
my white little lie. My earnest

endeavor drives on, do or die.
My thorough, throughout.

My easy was hard. My love & my life
for a crystalline shard. My pleasure,

whenever, to honor the sinner,
my mother & father & sister & killer.

Camus Reviewed by Smiley

killed almost is
reputation in the early

of his stranger paradoxes
when the boy

his son was reared
a brilliant an excellent time

he was married he was
21 a drug addict he yet

became thus wrote
& somewhat after was

to write again he was
in action called

formal belief & was
like his own absurd tradition

clearly years of family
has interest the book does not

set out to be pretend

After Borges

& here another alleyway
& here a sole groan

goes dead & here the local
folks & roped throats & here

the bright bird shits
histories all afternoon

& here tonight your light
makes mention

of a man amazed
by days (dopeless

hope fiend) (last junkie
standing) & here this

unknown anxious quick
thing (that's life)

After Stein

I have fellowshipped with sober
fellows. I have fellowshipped with

fellows who are not sober. I have
fellowshipped not sober with sober

fellows & fellows who are not. I have
sober fellowshipped with sobers who are

not fellows & I have fellowshipped
not sober with not sobers who nor

fellows neither sober are. Are not
today that on a sober day

I fellowshipped & fellowship
not sober not todays. Todays that is

& are I am to fellow sobers be.

Indelible in the Hippocampus

No, I don't much remember growing up.
If I remember rain, the rain

was always "pouring"—& days?
The sun did, or didn't, "shine."

An atrophy from infancy.
Days "go" like a river "flows,"

quickly, & altogether in a blur.
The rain starts ranting.

Over & over I tell myself
the story of my life.

Deep down, I do, I think,
want more than being found

at the wrong time of night
in the wrong part of town.

I'm about to drive in the ocean.
I'ma try to swim from something bigger than me.
Kick off my shoes and swim good.

FRANK OCEAN

Streaming Frank Ocean's Cover of "Moon River"

A slowness over stubborn plainscapes
in the total gain of water
from the flooded riverbed. As down
the grain by filigree a hat or bag
or basket weaves from straw unbundled
& reordered, so are you undone
& done again
by doctors' hands, which cursive
in your intimate apostrophes.
Such palomino lying in the rooms
of beige. Like golds unfolding
in a field among the tiny lives.

Streaming Rio Mangini's Cover of Chopin's "Ocean Étude"

Brother/fighter,
    time competes for you.

A child's rhyme,
    threadbare, barren beyond
our peers   even:

girls with thin curls
    were blond in black & white,

smoke   like fingers
    laying their heavy heads
to bed.

If I've earned a holiday,
    give me your Spain

from all four poles, your Portugal,
    a continent widening
in the belly of water.

Diving depths for rocks
    is a native danger, heretofore.

So tender a toreador.
    I have   not
worked all my life.

Streaming Queen's "Love of My Life" (Live at Rock in Rio)

Barefoot back & forth along the shore,
      the wind & waves make inalienable noise.

Together, they conspire against
          the wick in the basin of the sea.

      Blood plugs each ear.
        The tide is muted

    but strong, like hands grip a book
or bodies write cursive in sand.

Streaming Queen's "Somebody to Love"

the west will need no coastal alibi : the east is like a siren after finning
water bodies blot the plains : to endure the sun's romantic advances
or worse, to keep resisting hours : on end until it beds Pacific depths
a dry, extended fingertip : points Texas to Californ-I-A—I am
at stake in all of this : the thought of which
will (not) leave you : indifferent

Streaming Whitney Houston's "I Wanna Dance with Somebody"

A tide ablaze. Wood boats
discovered overturned & burned

where sand & sea
rocks snag beach debris

from floating to the bay.
It's distinctly 1960, hula parties

having gathered here,
though residents now claim

the shore for pets before
sunset. So much depends

upon a mind's leisure
& quick association.

Perhaps a skinny child was buried
to his neck in sand,

remade a merman
from Atlantis. Maybe waves

softened his scales to knees
& washed his thin arms free.

Remember me? The skinny limbs
remain unbothered.

The finest sands
can be reduced no farther.

Streaming Whitney Houston's "Queen of the Night"

If   a pessimist, if   under   water,

          can't   move myself,   can't   find a thing

to   move   me.   Fishes   are optimistic,

          fishes   swim   in   worship

                    through   the   heavy every   thing,

          covet a   goddess   who   deceives them

                    under   dancing   gold   strands.   A wig? A lie?

A myth?   If   I surface,   if   I turn   to   counting stars,

          would I   discern   what burns   the   unmixed   sky?

Streaming Robin Schlotz's Cover of Mozart's "Queen of the Night"

Of ambitions, Thoreau opined
we will only hit our aim.

Forgive us our paraphrases
(as we forgive those

who paraphrase against us):
to reach a height in failure,

we must intend to overshoot it.
Thorough Thoreau, advice

which does that very thing.
Although the rain, directionless,

has hit upon a new refrain,
from ice to water vapor.

So one lesson lacks ambition,
water's capacity for change.

Streaming Frank Ocean's "Nights"

On long delay, the falling sky
crashes Pacifically in tidal waves

off the wharf where beach commoners
must resist it. A ship ships

surplus cars & trucks
to water burial

deeper than souterrain,
under porpoises & water

mammals (no sirens per se,
or siren song's muted

by truck frame whirls & eddies).
Decades hence, there's word

of car part afterlives.
The shipman's grandson dreamt

dreams through his father's
father, who slid machinery to sea,

where it awoke as from a slumber,
took female form, & sang

to forlorn shipmen of the day.
In this (as in his every dream)

a captive seal dies & lies like metal
on the zoo pool's cement floor,

six thousand copper-plated weights
gorged to gut-burst. Might

as well a plane wing splitting
the Pacific shallows with its arc,

sunlit pennies set off
like underwater sparks.

Thank god I have an innocent eye for nature.

PETER ORLOVSKY

Music Theory

Fall's folding. Congeries of leaves
are finished filling out, leaving.
The vinyl street breaks off
with no returns at 43rd.
Tomorrow's the same song,
though every moment
modifies a note.
No diatonic shift
should steady time's beat so,
instead should only notice
what occurs, intone it.
If I say it is, it is.
I have an ear for this.

Original Motion Picture Soundtrack

The moon melon ripens
on the horizon. A road opens
trafficless under watch
of triangle tower lights,
apartment windows
bright like TVs
lining the empty streets.
We drive around downtown,
the inner burbs,
ignore what whirs
inside the car
(we're stars)
because the camera's far
& blurs particulars.
Lowering the radio,
songs blend into a warm hum.
Smiles signal the scene
is brief. (A beat.)
The burden is to speak
or fade away. To hum along.
To memorize my line, then say:

After Chopin's "Wrong Note Étude"

I've been
at your window.
to throw. Broken
the breeze
Some fingers feel
like liquid drying.
to be the finger
the verb that does
but push. This, too:
the bird in the bush
Or both? To take
with wingless

something
Something
inside,
still blows.
cold on skin,
I'd like that:
that points,
nothing in crisis
to be
or the hand.
the wind
willingness.

Ode to Nancy Reagan

Homebound, morning mirrors
yesterday, sun lighting
a hand stencil of REVOLUTION
on the cracked concrete.
My bike tire strikes it.
I was told a story once
in school, how no Soviet
would be the first
to halt applause & sit.
Downhill & to the right
a bat circles the street
with the squeak
of loose axles or unhinged
metal parts, each flutter
on the broken blue like two
hands stopping short of clap.

After Chopin's "Revolutionary Étude"

Windy involvements
scuffle down & down for miles
like black-backed birds
mistaken for upward forces
not meant to form
this bruiseface afternoon
from distant virga:
wisped too slight for splash
in shadows that play
across the horizontal plains,
as spring recalls to follow
winter—winter, fall—as fledging
swallows know by nature
or some other thing than learning
to hold a second destination in the will.

Carillon Cento

Hour (a plunge)
on hour (a lark),
the tower bells bedew
the waking remnants
in this isle of men,
dear land of flesh-
kept creaturehood.
A stubbornly embodied
donkey drinks the useful,
lowly water many times
from many streams
which flow for months
untouched, as a tree
lets winds run up & down
its branches, singing.
The sound of an ancient spring
nulls the donkey's bray.
Like an elderly embrace
(slow enough, too long)
the thorough bells anticipate.
"Fear no more,"
yells the bell embodied.

Prelude to Retrocast

First words overheard are savory
conversation, "violin" & "instrument,"
a woman's mouth still marking them.
I recall a childhood day like today,
wind rousing leaves in static pitches,
the connotation of the storm
worse than the storm. What rains
might come of it? What sudden floods?
It suffices to send people
into houses & government buildings.
We brave rain mists, the wind
trilling, failing to make more of itself.
Its gusts a "sinfonia," she's overheard
to say. The tree above her forks
three ways. The largest branch
begins to play a creak near breaking.
Like crickets in the million violinning.

The Recognizable Difference Between Notes

An ambulance premeditates
among some numbered impossibilities,
which all the world's
behavior seconds & approves.
Keeping to himself,
his distaste for taste proliferates.
Though recognizable, flowers
are anything but floral,
another case of parts, together,
amounting to the less-than-ideal.
The streets are safe & soundless.
(To say there is no sound
implies, also, a want of music.)
No sooner does he notice this,
the violin against the brick
produces notes he notices
in intervals of fifths.

Continuous Burlesk

Breezes bare a hairline. Small leaves
blotch the gentleman's hand
like age. In the city, his mind
was lit in neon. Now memory
persists in a small flowering.
There are no mirrors
in the hotel room,
but many metal doors.
Deep in the chest of the other man
is a fist. The TV (like a fist)
is mute. Brigitte Bardot
has hardened, but, younger
once, danced French ballet.
Her feet formed fists.
Is nature's noise a happy song?
Dance strings the afternoon
with asterisks.

One day this kid will
come to know something that causes a sensation
equivalent to the separation of the earth from
its axis. One day this kid will reach a point
where he senses a division that isn't
mathematical.

DAVID WOJNAROWICZ

Red Menace

        on high   our robin
           is the first
spring   bud to bloom

hung there
        among the   trees
like   broken glass

catching   light & rain
             drops
trucks

      don't slow   for him
   too small   to cut
         bicycles   ride

      right past
   wing beats like spokes
      on playing cards   (the Red King)

      dirt predator
softly stalking
        rhubarb   corridors

for small
      treasure
mischief in bushes   is his

he plays the worm game   alone

Color Theory

After my brother & his friends dye the eggs
their blues & greens & pinks, they press

Snoopy stickers over light blotches & cracks
where the dye won't take.

That's what all my family does
on Easter since I'm gone. They sit

(not talking) & press stickers
where the color never seems to want to go.

Rods & Cones

Given horses, I learn to ride
from my mistakes, men spreading

in the kicks of dirt. To mount
before the others, early sun grasping

over hills. Light like a wrist, light like a rib,
light like the fresh green fingers of sod.

To shade the shed with my run,
sight blurring its all-too-quick, too-big.

To ride past those who can't say "no"
when "yes" suffices. To find "yes"

feels quite right & lie awake inside
the dream. To think, I thought

the earth had almost broke apart.
To trust the ground is sometimes held

together by a single root of grass.

Hayden loved to climb to the summit on one of the barren hills flanking the river, & stand there while the wind blew

syllables & sighs. Oh, the sounds around
us were just words (a warren
of warnings) & flowed like argot.

Grandma was said to say, "a hitch
in my get-along," conveying many things
(a love of horseback) (life is a rough

ride). Despite all we were
led to believe we could neither lead
the horse nor make it drink.

Oh, the river bends but (oh)
it rarely breaks so ("hell or high
water") let's go in & do our work.

Would the clock never strike? Nerves were snapping, but Hayden gave no hint of it

Whereas we enter
& choose a chair (the paradox
of chairs is to calculate

& not divide the room). Join in,
won't you, & forego the gutter
view? Unseat yourself

from the cement. Eye skies
pocked by radar blips. Good vibes
lengthen intervals of dips.

We listen when lips loosen.
We outlast shouts.
We pander, ply, & plead.

Poor Pandora, please
subject yourself & stop unlocking.
Can't math make us match?

Integer to integer (whole
numbers humming under)
ever to unbox the room.

Looking longingly into the brown eyes of Hayden the Unattainable

Who, here,
positions himself perpendicular
to a glance? (Some say

a glance could be
a wince.) (Some say
every man has his autumn.)

Is this the season yearned for,
yet unearned? (Some say,
instead of "autumn," "fall.")

Is this feeling (recursive
& erased) a draft?
(Some say inside his eyes

the photons of galaxies
pertain.) So much
(some say) can go unsaid.

Go, Hayden, & that right speedily

Follow that lad, as one does a feather,
not on foot (or so much by sight) (don't stray)
but by imagination. We have here

a failure to commit to memory
& follow through. What floods the mind
are adages I never learned (never mind
the words I wrote & stow away).

I feel for you (here, among my upper
ribs) & better uncage it. As curtains clip the day,
winter differs so little from a summer

night, except Orion in his corner of the sky.
I telescope & I refract my find.
I ruminate on seasons & (in kind)
remark the ways of water. (Do I reach to say

Earth's waters are equally the Moon's?) Four
horizons reframe the sky. Rhyme is shiny-
minded & bite-sized. Rhyme reaches from behind.

After Jane Hammond, *Untitled*, 1991

(Unlike a) helicopter
doors) helicopter
(& "pteron" for some
my head (the mind
doors to many dreams)
a bat) (like a hooded
but younger

(the human mind
(from "helix" for "spiral")
thing that feels like a touch
has no image for absence)
(cornered) I see a color
garment) (soft like
once danced

has no metal
(not "helio" for "sun")
or twirl) over
(the absent mind has
& the color is blind (like
fur) (I have hardened
Russian ballet).

Not last night but
(close to calling it
at my door (sweet
what they want
Spanish dancer
give a high (five)
Spanish dancer turn
dancer (close enough
Spanish dancer run (me

(half past) the (mid)night
quits cold turkey)
surrender) (nevermore)
& this (in turn) is
do the splits
(take the high road) (sink or
(that cheek) around (now
to) touch (the sky
ragged in my home) (now

before 24 robbers came
(who's that) knocking
I asked them
what they said:
Spanish dancer
swim, both are a) kick
the other cheek) Spanish
& grasp) the ground
get the flip) out of town.

Cinderella
& shoes
to a quiet request)
her mistake (the grand
escape) she kissed
many (shoes in a
hard to get) (oh

(could be depressed)
of corresponding)
went upstairs to kiss a
entrance mistook itself
a snake (charmer) (handler)
funeral procession fit or
dear) doctors

dressed in (a dress
yellow (responding
(requiting) fellow
for the emergency
(oil salesman) how
floats in a parade play
did it take?

After Christopher Wool, *Untitled*, 1991

un be k now nst a st ash
un der the rug   a reg
ular   abomi nat i on

on ly   a car to   on   mi rage
or st raw to break the came l
out back be hind the slid ing frame

if th is   point an dc lick fame
is raz or jaw or in stag ram par
iah (par cel & par ty) towhat

ex tent do I o wet his pleas an try?
even tu ally   y'all enter   an
even ing al read y ren de red

all road s con verge to reg u late
a reg   u lar   ab dom   in
al & all   the   for est ss urge

After Félix González-Torres, *Untitled*, 1991

Some mornings I see a tree
limb flexing outside the thin glass
& can all but hear its branches
juggle the leaves. How some wind loves
to tickle, countless seeds
giggling in accomplishment.

Some mornings in the thin glass
a bright saltwater fish sees me wait
outside the blood draw filling
my chair with wiggles.
Silent, the scientist sees
my blood mingle on the thin glass
as air conditions the room
like a morning breeze.

Despite all risk, how some love winds
up full frontal, filling the walls
with struggle. Somehow
love wins & leaves
its countless empty beds
like trophies around town.

After David Wojnarowicz, *Untitled (Face in Dirt)*, 1991

The sand (frets) underfoot. Feet over (reach) the beach.
The planks (split) in the pier. Some grains (grind) in the teeth.

The gritty (clenched) smile of the giddy (firstborn) child.
A slim beginner (swimmer's) summer to while.

The softwood (is known for) needles. The hardwood (for) leaves.
The lips learn (to shape) a dozen ways to (say) please.

I fit any body part (& depart) with personal style.
Fall really got me gone (all along) meanwhile.

The bike (spoke) on glazed flakes, a rod in the (split) wrist.
A Jesus who Saves. (Fatboy Slim at a rave.) I don't make the list.

Art hangs (like tombstones) in each pupil on the Miracle Mile.
Picture perfect (movie trailer) winter weather all the while.

Where (one asks) lives the whisper, in the throat or the ear?
Where (one answers) lives forever, in a moment, over years.

The doctor, the healer, the (art) dealer, this (s)inner child.
Look around (spring has sprung), lie back down, stay awhile.

Notes

This collection is also dedicated to the memory of two dear poetry teachers: Jake Adam York & Thomas Whitbread.

"Feedback Loop" quotes Lil Wayne's 2008 song "A Milli."

"Habits of Creature" takes its refrain from Marcel Dzama's 2014 painting *My mother, my father, my sister, my killer, my lover, my savior, and other faces I once knew.*

"Camus Reviewed by Smiley" is an erasure poem from a newspaper review of the biography *Albert Camus: A Life.*

"After Borges" alludes to & loosely translates his poem "Texas."

"After Stein" alludes to a passage from *The Autobiography of Alice B. Toklas.*

The title "Indelible in the Hippocampus" is from Christine Blasey Ford's September 27, 2018, Senate Judicial Committee testimony.

"Streaming Frank Ocean's Cover of 'Moon River'" is for Dheya.

"Streaming Rio Mangini's Cover of Chopin's 'Ocean Étude'" is for Dean. Mangini was a piano prodigy whose childhood performances are viewable on YouTube.

Then-14-year-old Robin Schlotz's performance of Mozart's "Queen of the Night" is viewable on YouTube.

"Carillon Cento" is composed of interleaved phrases from St. Francis of Assisi & Virginia Woolf.

"Rods & Cones" is for Janko.

The titles "Hayden loved to climb to the summit on one of the barren hills flanking the river, & stand there while the wind blew," "Would the clock never strike? Nerves were snapping, but Hayden gave no hint of it," "Looking longingly into the brown eyes of Hayden the Unattainable," & "Go, Hayden, &

that right speedily" are adapted from four painting titles by N.C. Wyeth.

"Hayden loved to climb to the summit on one of the barren hills flanking the river, & stand there while the wind blew" is dedicated to the memory of my grandparents, Pat Carey, Elaine Lambert, & Robert Lambert.

"After Jane Hammond, *Untitled*, 1991" quotes three jump rope rhymes. The painting is on view in my bedroom.

Untitled, 1991, by Christopher Wool is sometimes on view at MoMA & is viewable online.

Untitled, 1991, by Félix González-Torres was billboarded all over American towns during the height of the AIDS pandemic & is also viewable online.

Untitled (Face in Dirt), 1991, was David Wojnarowicz's final authorized work & is viewable online.

The epigraph "One must imagine Sisyphus happy" is from Blaise Pascal's 1942 essay, *Le Mythe de Sisyphe (The Myth of Sisyphus)*.

The epigraph "It was a night" is widely attributed to a French interview with Brigitte Bardot.

The epigraph from Frank Ocean's "Swim Good" is reprinted by permission of Hal Leonard LLC. Words & Music by Christopher Breaux, Waynne Nugent, Kevin Risto, & Charlie Gambetta. Copyright © 2010 Heavens Research, Sony Music Publishing LLC, Waynne Writers & Break North Music. All rights for Heavens Research Administered by BMG Rights Management (US) LLC. All rights for Sony Music Publishing LLC, Waynne Writers, & Break North Music Administered by Sony Music Publishing LLC, 424 Church Street, Suite 1200, Nashville, TN 37219. All rights reserved & used by permission.

Peter Orlovsky's epigraph is from his 1957 "Second Poem." The poem appeared in Orlovsky's out-of-print *Clean Asshole Poems and Smiling Vegetable Songs* & is now widely available online.

The final epigraph by David Wojnarowicz is from in his 1991 photostat print *Untitled (One day this kid)* & is viewable online.

Acknowledgements

I so appreciate the editors & publications who first published these poems, often as different iterations or under alternate titles:

Borderlands: Texas Poetry Review	After Chopin's "Revolutionary Étude"
Copper Nickel	Prelude to Retrocast
Crab Creek Review	After David Wojnarowicz, *Untitled (Face in Dirt)*, 1991
Crab Creek Review	Feedback Loop
Crab Creek Review	Mr. Liquor Delivers
CutBank: All Accounts & Mixture	Rods & Cones
Denver Quarterly	After Félix González-Torres, *Untitled*, 1991
Denver Quarterly	After Jane Hammond, *Untitled*, 1991
Harpur Palate	Red Menace
Harpur Palate	Streaming Frank Ocean's "Nights"
Harpur Palate	Streaming Rio Mangini's Cover of Chopin's "Ocean Étude"
Kelp Journal	Streaming Queen's "Love of My Life" (Live at Rock in Rio)
Kelp Journal	Streaming Whitney Houston's "I Wanna Dance with Somebody"
Kelp Journal	Streaming Whitney Houston's "Queen of the Night"
New Letters	Habits of Creature
Oddball Magazine	Color Theory
peculiar: a queer literary journal	After Stein
Río Grande Review	*Music Theory*
Superstition Review	Fight, Flight, Freeze
Superstition Review	The Recognizable Difference Between Notes
Temenos	Future Tense
Temenos	Ode to Nancy Reagan
Tupelo Quarterly	Continuous Burlesk
Tupelo Quarterly	Hayden loved to climb to the summit on one of the barren hills flanking the river, & stand there while the wind blew
The Worcester Review	Indelible in the Hippocampus
Yalobusha Review	After Christopher Wool, *Untitled*, 1991

Special Thanks

I'm most indebted to my family for rocket launches & soft landings: Bonny, Dad, Mom, Kip, Dean, Cristina, & Georgia. Thank you for standing by me in belief.

I'm grateful, as well, to my friends for soft launches & rocket landings: Nicholas Ong, Chris Pollock, Hayden Hunt, Louis W. Tullius, Patrick Gray, Scott William Ward, James Barry, Christopher Melchi, Larry, Kevin, Berenice, Harriet, Dheya, Chris K., Randall, Beth, Lucía, Lisa, Natalia, & Janko.

This collection & my poetry have benefitted from the support of Jessica Piazza, James Capozzi, Math Trafton, Jeffrey Wolf, Gina Anderson-Lopez, Derek Robbins, Cate Wiley, Michael Henry, The University of Texas at Austin (especially David Wevill & Kurt Heinzelman), & the Michener Center for Writers (especially Marie Howe & Naomi Shihab Nye).

Thank you to everyone at Finishing Line Press for bringing this book into the light—thank you to two of my favorite poets, Mary Ann Samyn & Justin Jannise, for your bright blurbs—& thank you to Loui Jover for your mind-blowing cover art.

Finally, I thank my MUSC friends & colleagues for sharing in my successes: Jennie Ariail, Michelle Cohen, John Dinolfo, Christy Huggins, Lisa Kerr, Casey O'Neill, & Tom Smith.

R.J. Lambert (he, him, his) grew up near Denver and survived the 1999 Columbine High School shootings in Littleton, Colorado. He has since been interested in how individuals and communities respond to crises—relationship violence, environmental disasters, mental health, and HIV/AIDS—through writing.

As one of the first alumni of the undergraduate writing program at the University of Colorado at Denver, R.J. co-founded the student literary journal that would become *Copper Nickel* with fellow students and the late poet Jake Adam York. As a graduate student and Michener Fellow at the University of Texas at Austin, he co-founded and co-edited the literary journal *Bat City Review* along with poets Jessica Piazza, James Capozzi, and Kurt Heinzelman.

R.J.'s poetry has been featured in numerous print and online venues, including the forthcoming anthology *Without a Doubt* (New York Quarterly Press). His poem "Habits of Creature" was chosen by Kaveh Akbar to receive the 2021 Patricia Cleary Miller Award for Poetry from *New Letters,* and *The Worcester Review* nominated "Indelible in the Hippocampus" for a Pushcart Prize. Other poems were published finalists for the *Tupelo Quarterly* Broadside Prize and the *Crab Creek Review* Poetry Prize. This is his debut poetry collection.

R.J. also holds a doctorate in Rhetoric and Composition from the University of Texas at El Paso. He has presented and published research on failed crisis responses to ecological disasters, teaching and learning during extreme situations, diversity and cancel culture, queer representation in contemporary literature, and the poetry and poetics of HIV/AIDS.

Having worked for many years in cancer research as a medical editor and grant writer at the University of Washington School of Medicine in Seattle, R.J. now teaches scientific and professional writing as an Assistant Professor in the Center for Academic Excellence & Writing Center at the Medical University of South Carolina. Within the MUSC Office of Humanities, he regularly assists with courses offerings, humanities events, and outreach programs, such as MUSC's annual statewide Septima P. Clark Student Poetry Competition.

CPSIA information can be obtained
at www.ICGtesting.com
Printed in the USA
BVHW041938160822
644725BV00016B/208

9 781646 628230